Teeth Whitening Cure:

Natural Teeth Whitening At Home

By Gordon Stevens

CONTENTS

CHAPTER 1:
INTRODUCTION

Teeth can become stained and discolored from years of drinking coffee, soda, or tea, or from smoking. Fluoride treatments can also cause teeth to develop a motley series of spots and splotches

Despite the fact that teeth whitening is primarily cosmetic, most individuals with white teeth also have healthy teeth, which is why the two go hand in hand. Finding the perfect teeth whitener and getting into a constant routine is the only way to achieve that sparkling smile. Discover what we recommend for the whitest teeth possible below.

If you're looking for an effective at-home teeth whitening methods, I have good news for you – I will reveal all the insider secrets to getting a perfect smile at a fraction of what you would pay elsewhere.

In the past few decades, dental hygiene has become more of a center-point for overall health. We now understand that a lot of health
related problems can be cut off before they even start, by keeping on top of brushing , flossing and taking care of our teeth. Most people that have a sparkling smile make a strong effort to take care of their teeth more than once a day. One of the most important aspects of sporting a gleaming, white smile is being in a constant routine and using the correct techniques to really make your teeth glow. You can't expect perfect teeth without giving daily effort.

Below, I'll take you through how to take care of your teeth, what makes up a daily routine and how to get your teeth to shine with the right whitener.

UNDERSTANDING YOUR TEETH

To fully understand the best way to take care of our teeth, let's take a look back at how teeth start off. In early childhood, our teeth are completely covered by very strong, porcelain-like enamel that acts as a protective barrier. Due to the daily stress we put our teeth; this enamel slowly wears away, becoming more translucent. This permits the yellow color of dentin (the tooth's core material) to show through, giving your teeth that dingy, unappealing look. Due to constant chewing, millions of micro-cracks can also occur over the years. These cracks easily get filled up with excess debris, allowing stains to form and potentially
causing cavities. Taking care of your teeth, as well as using the proper teeth whitening techniques, can help remove this plague build-up and the stains associated with the wear-and-tear of your daily eating routine.

Take a second to think of what passes
through your mouth in a single day. On average, at least 3-4 meals of food, anything you drink or snack on. How many times have you been too tired at night to pick yourself up to get into the bathroom and give your teeth a brush? We're all guilty of it, but if you want a whiter, healthier smile, breaking that habit and brushing is one of the key components.

GETTING INTO A CONSTANT ROUTINE

Let's be real straight up about this: taking care of your teeth is a never ending process. Just like shaving and taking showers, it's an activity you'll have to do daily if you want that beautiful, white smile. This is a lifestyle change you'll have to make for yourself. We're not saying you'll need to be in the bathroom brushing constantly, or punish yourself if you miss a day or two, but a continual effort is necessary.

To adequately take care of your teeth, it's best to run through your teeth regimen after breakfast and before going to bed, sometime after dinner. This allows your teeth to be clean most of the day and while you sleep, two big chunks of the average person's life.

A RECOMMENDED TEETH WHITENING & CLEANING REGIMEN

Again, it's suggested to use this regimen once after breakfast, before you start your day and once after dinner, before you go to sleep. This will take about 30-40 extra minutes a day, so allow a little bit of time to adjust. Once you're in the routine, it'll be a piece of cake and the results will come quickly.

1 - Start off by using a home treatment, for the suggested time, which is usually 5-10 minutes. I prefer using this first, so you can brush off the excess whitener that is left on your teeth and gums. (I'll go into more detail later, including a full review about which whitening product I highly recommend).
2 - Next, use an electric tooth brush, to generously clean all of your teeth. This includes the front, underside and back. Don't forget to give your tongue a good scrubbing, too.
3 - Grab a flossing tool (which is easier to manage than actual floss) and take some time to clean in-between each of your teeth. This is a target area for cavities to begin, since food and grime tends to build up easily in there, also causing stains in-between your teeth.
4 - As a final step, rinse with a mouth wash product to help protect and keep your teeth clean until the next time you brush. This also gives you extra minty, fresh breath, which is always a

plus. A good option is using LISTERINE MOUTH WASH. It is inexpensive and does the work, plus you totally get rid of bad breath which is very important if you engage in conversations and want others to stay close.

To give yourself an added dose of whiteness, I highly recommend using a teeth whitening product everyday that you brush. This will help boost the white shades of your teeth to an even greater level. We've personally tried almost every product offered on the market over the years, but as technology advances, the old whiteners lose their effectiveness, making room for easier to use, more efficient products.

Teeth Whitening AT THE COMFORT OF YOUR HOME

I really don't want you to spend a dime more than you have to in order to have a white smile. So I am going to show you can do everything at home, using everyday ingredients and still get amazing results. No expensive stuff, no 55$ special mouthwash...cheap affordable things you probably already have at home right now.

CHAPTER 2: EVERYTHING YOU NEED TO KNOW ABOUT TEETH WHITENING

Stained or yellowish teeth are a common cosmetic concern but there are many different options for removing superficial or intrinsic stains. Before you make a decision about whitening, weigh your options and consider the pros and cons of professional services versus at-home pastes or kits.

FDA REGULATION

According to the Food and Drug Administration, teeth "whitening" refers to any procedure that restores teeth to their natural color by removing stains. The FDA defines "bleaching" as any process that whitens teeth beyond their natural color. The FDA does not regulate whitening products, so you should consult your dentist before using whiteners.

STAINS

Dental stains are either extrinsic or intrinsic. Extrinsic stains are superficial and are caused by coffee, tea or soda consumption; smoking, foods and daily wear and tear. Extrinsic stains can usually be eliminated with at-home whitening treatments or by dental cleanings. Intrinsic stains occur on the interior of the teeth and result from excessive fluoride exposure, aging, trauma or exposure to certain minerals during development. According to the Consumer Guide to Dentistry, extrinsic stains are more difficult to remove, but supervised, long-term use of at-home whiteners can make a difference.

TOOTHPASTE

According to Alan Carr, D.M.D., whitening toothpastes can help to eliminate surface stains caused by coffee consumption or smoking. These toothpastes include fine abrasives that polish the surface of the teeth and chemicals that dissolve stains. They generally take several weeks to work and will not

change the natural color of your teeth. Although whitening pastes are usually safe for daily use, excessive use can damage your enamel. Dr. Carr recommends that you look for the American Dental Association Seal of Approval on the paste to ensure its safety.

PROFESSIONAL WHITENING

Most dentists offer in-office bleaching procedures. The advantage of professional whitening is that your dentist will take every precaution to protect your teeth and gums, and the results should be apparent immediately. The disadvantage of professional whitening is that it can be expensive.

AT HOME

Your dentist may offer take-home bleach kits as an alternative to office whitening. The take-home kits are less expensive and include a peroxide gel that is left on the teeth for about an hour.

You can also purchase over-the- counter kits at a local pharmacy. While professional kits use hydrogen peroxide as the primary active ingredient, over-the-counter kits use carbamide peroxide which has about 1/3 the strength of the professional kits. Over-the-counter kits, although less expensive, may be less effective and take longer to work.

RISKS

Whitening and bleaching procedures can result in a temporary sensitivity to temperature and sweetness. Although the sensitivity only lasts a few days, you may want to invest in a toothpaste for sensitive teeth following the procedure. Additionally, peroxide whiteners can cause inflammation and irritation of the gums. Whitening may result in an unexpected cosmetic disadvantage. Since crowns, veneers and bonding do not respond to whiteners, your teeth may whiten unevenly

CHAPTER 3: HOW TO WHITEN YOUR TEETH AT HOME

HOW CAN YOU GET WHITER TEETH FOR FREE?

Don't spend your hard-earned money on expensive teeth whitening kits! Get the very same results absolutely free. Don't pay a high office call to go to the dentist and get your teeth professionally whitened! You can have white teeth with things that are probably just sitting in your medicine chest or kitchen cupboard. Don't bother with those gel packs that you have to leave on your teeth. Don't buy that expensive mouthwash for smokers! You have everything that you need to brighten and whiten your teeth right in your own home. Remember that this is free and it works.

DO I HAVE THESE ITEMS IN MY HOUSE?

All you need to whiten your teeth are simple household products. Ok, first go to the kitchen. Open the cupboard where you keep your baking supplies. Do you have baking soda? You probably do. Spoon about two teaspoons of baking soda into a little bowl or cup. Now, travel over to the nearest bathroom. Open the medicine chest. Do you have hydrogen peroxide? You probably have this common household item, too.

Whitening your teeth does not have to be expensive. In fact, home remedies provide a successful way to get whiter teeth without spending a fortune on a trip to the dentist, or on an over-the-counter whitening kit. Using natural products to whiten teeth can take a bit longer than high-tech lasers and bleaching lights, but you will have peace of mind knowing that what you are using is safe.

THE SECRET TO WHITE TEETH? SUPER STRONG ELEMENTS!

Let Me specify a bit about the different available elements you may choose to use for Whitening your Teeth. On the next section, we will mix them up to make a very powerful paste.

#1: HYDROGEN PEROXIDE

Many over-the-counter tooth-whitening remedies contain hydrogen peroxide. Tufts University reports that hydrogen peroxide penetrates the enamel and dentin layers of your teeth, producing free radicals that ultimately create single-carbon bonds. These single-carbon bonds reflect light, and make teeth look whiter.
Pour a few teaspoons of hydrogen peroxide into a bathroom cup, and dip your toothbrush inside. Brush your teeth with the hydrogen peroxide for two minutes, rinsing with water afterward. Apply the hydrogen peroxide once a day, between normal brushings, for best results.

The process goes as follows:

STEP 1:

Brush your teeth normally, with regular toothpaste. Rinse thoroughly with water. Set the toothpaste and toothbrush aside.

STEP 2:

Pour a small quantity of peroxide, less than 1/4 cup, into a fresh rinsing glass. Swish it around the entire mouth for approximately 1 minute, being careful not to swallow any of the peroxide (gargling is safe, as long as no liquid enters your throat). Spit it into the sink and rinse it down the drain (peroxide

left anywhere, including on porcelain, immediately begins a bleaching and cleaning process that can be heard in the form of a hissing of small bubbles frothing up).

STEP 3:

As an alternative or in addition to rinsing and spitting, dip a clean cotton swab into the peroxide and rub it along the tooth surfaces. This technique cannot get into the spaces between teeth, but it can be useful to increase the whitening of visible surfaces.

STEP 4:

Rinse thoroughly with plain water, taking as long as a minute again to completely rinse the peroxide out of your mouth. Spit it into the sink and, again, rinse the sink with water. If bubbles are felt fizzing between or around the teeth, rinse again until the peroxide is completely removed.

STEP 5:

Repeat daily (results are typically seen in 2 weeks or less). After an acceptable degree of whitening has been achieved, discontinue daily peroxide use in favor of weekly sessions.

TIPS AND WARNINGS

According to the American Dental Association (ADA), it is safe to use peroxide to whiten teeth. You may feel some burning in your gums while swishing with peroxide, but this is not harmful. The ADA recommends consulting with a dentist before beginning a home tooth- whitening program, especially for people with dark stains on their teeth, crowns or many fillings.

Be careful not to splash any peroxide onto clothes, towels or dark painted surfaces, since the peroxide can bleach the color out of these

in spots. Use of peroxide can cause some tooth sensitivity or irritation of your gums.

#2: BAKING SODA

Meet your new best friend. Baking soda is non-toxic and has been used for many years for a variety of cleaning purposes. It is also effective for cleaning and whitening teeth. Bonus--it kills germs in your mouth that can cause plaque.

Baking soda helps maintain an internal acidity balance, and has a variety of uses, including cleaning, extinguishing fires, and polishing teeth. This gentle abrasive forms from soda ash and works well as a stain-removing agent. Pour a few teaspoons of baking soda into a bathroom cup, and dip your damp toothbrush into it. Brush your teeth with the baking soda for two minutes, rinsing afterward with water. Because baking soda is an abrasive, you should only brush with it two to three times a week.

Baking soda has a myriad of household uses as well as providing various health benefits, including the benefit of whitening teeth. Known as sodium bicarbonate, the substance is found in mineral springs or can easily be produced artificially.

HOW DOES BAKING SODA WORK?

Mildly alkaline, baking soda dissolves in water in order to penetrate tooth enamel. With a slightly abrasive action, the free radicals that are emitted once baking soda is mixed in water help to scrape off the yellow or brown stains that buildup from drinking coffee, tea, colas or from smoking or chewing

tobacco. In this way, the mixture is able to break down discoloration as it interacts with stain molecules to lighten and brighten teeth.

OTHER BENEFITS OF USING BAKING SODA

Baking soda also removes plaque, helping to prevent tooth decay and to freshen the breath. As one of the least expensive substances on the market, using baking soda is a great way to avoid spending money on commercial teeth whitening kits or thousands of dollars on in-office whitening treatments.

HOW TO BRUSH WITH BAKING SODA

Cleaning your teeth with baking soda is as easy as it is with regular toothpaste. Just dampen your toothbrush and dip it into a small pile of baking soda, making sure to cover all the bristles.

Brush your teeth for two minutes, making sure to reach each and every tooth. Once you are done with this thorough brushing, spit out the excess baking soda and then rinse your mouth with water. If you feel a burning or tingling sensation, this is normal as the baking soda performs its cleaning action. If you want to add extra whitening power, wet your toothbrush with hydrogen peroxide instead of water and then dip into the baking soda.

Do not brush your teeth with baking soda more than once a week. More frequent brushing can cause the enamel coating on your teeth to become damaged. Be careful not to brush too hard for the same reason. Use regular toothpaste for all other brushings, which should be a minimum of twice daily (morning and night) and after each meal.

Do not brush with baking soda if you use orthodontic glue or if you have braces or wear a permanent retainer.

#3: STRAWBERRIES

Yes, that's right – Strawberries. Not only are strawberries good for your health, they are also good for your teeth. In fact, Health.com notes that strawberries provide a quick and inexpensive way to whiten your teeth. Malic acid, a natural enzyme in strawberries, creates the whitening action. You can whiten with strawberries several ways, including by rubbing the ripe fruit on your teeth, or eating the strawberries and allowing the malic acid to sit on your teeth for five to 10 minutes as it removes stains. A final alternative is to mash a ripe strawberry in a small bowl using a fork. Mix in half a teaspoon of baking soda, and apply the strawberry mixture to a toothbrush. Brush for five minute and rinse. Follow up with a second brushing using regular toothpaste. Brush with strawberries once a week.

#4: WATER

Sometimes, the simplest solutions get overlooked. Simply rinses your mouth as soon as possible after eating may go a long way in preventing coffee, sodas and other staining agents from lingering in the mouth. According to Sid Kirchheimer in "The Doctors Book of Home Remedies II,"
even the simple act of discreetly swishing water in your mouth before swallowing makes a big difference when you can't get to a restroom to rinse or brush your teeth.

#5: SAGE LEAVES

I definitely recommends this old-fashioned quick tooth-whitening remedy that can be done in the great outdoors. Simply taking a sage leaf from your herb garden and wiping it over teeth and gums may make
them brighter because of sage's astringent properties. Alternatively, dry and grind sage leaves for use as a tooth powder, or infuse fresh leaves and rinse with the cooled, strained water.

#6: LEMON

Lemon juice is a commonly suggested method for whitening your teeth without having to resort to over-the- counter chemical tooth whiteners
.Unfortunately, the acid in lemon juice can damage your teeth.

The recommended method is to brush your teeth with lemon juice. This is not a recommended procedure as the acid in lemon juice will dissolve enamel over time. In the short term it can also make teeth extremely sensitive.

Beware, Lemon juice contains citric acid. When you apply lemon juice to your teeth, it erodes the enamel on the surface of the teeth. This may temporarily remove stains. But over time, the acid may erode the enamel until it exposes the yellow dentin underneath. The teeth may become sensitive to hot and cold temperatures or to certain kinds of foods. If you choose to use lemon juice to whiten your teeth, be sure to rinse the juice off after brushing and don't do it frequently. I would advise consulting your dentist before using Lemon juice.

#7: Whitening Foods

Adding certain foods to your diet may make an effective tool in your arsenal of natural tooth-whiteners. I would recommend crunchy foods like apples and celery to knock away food particles. Opinions vary on the classic lemon juice rinse for quick tooth whitening. Griggs includes it in her list of effective home remedies, but Grannymed.com warns that even occasional use of the acidic fruit may harm tooth enamel.

#8: Other Remedies

Brush with apple cider vinegar for 5 minutes before brushing with normal toothpaste.

Eat fresh vegetables and rub them over your teeth while chewing. Naturally-abrasive vegetables include celery, unpeeled carrots, broccoli and unpeeled cucumbers. Don't do this in front of dinner guests.

CHAPTER 4: THE SECRET ULTRA-PASTE THAT WILL MAKE YOUR TEETH SHINE!

Here is my ultimate paste which helps make your teeth super white, the natural way. This paste allows you to fully utilize the benefits of each of the above ingredients, and overall makes it so much easier to implement for you every day Whitening regimen (as a substitute for your plain toothpaste).

HOW DO I MAKE THIS PASTE?

Drop two or three teaspoons (this may not be exact) of the hydrogen peroxide into the baking soda, making a paste. This sometimes takes a little trial and error. Be sure it is the same consistency as toothpaste. If you wish, you can add a bit of mint flavoring or even a small dollop of toothpaste.

HOW DO I USE THIS FREE WHITENER?

Brush your teeth with your mixture, being sure to leave it on your teeth for at least two minutes. Do NOT swallow this paste! Trust me, you wouldn't want to swallow it- the taste is not the best. To make the paste taste better, try to use the above tips. This will help to make the taste a little bit tastier.

WHAT SHOULD I DO AFTER USING THIS PASTE?

After you finish brushing with this free paste, brush again with regular toothpaste to rid your mouth of the taste as well as the peroxide solution. You will be amazed at just how white and bright your teeth will be! Many smokers and heavy coffee drinkers use this little trick. This may be a home remedy that your grandmother even used.

I have a dental condition. Should I try this whitener? Beware that if you have open sores, cavities, gingivitis, or other gum diseases this may make your gums appear white for a short time. This may not be the whitener for your teeth if they are very sensitive. As with anything, you should consult your dentist before trying this or any other medical treatment.

HOW OFTEN CAN I USE THIS PASTE?

This treatment can be done weekly, monthly, or whenever you want extra bright teeth!

You shouldn't brush with this mixture more than once per week.

List of Items Needed:

- 3 teaspoons of hydrogen peroxide (the amount may vary depending on family size)
- 2 teaspoons of baking soda (the amount may vary depending on family size)
- Optional (A small amount of toothpaste or drop of mint flavor may also be added.)

This easy process will put a bright smile on your face!

Chapter 4: Natural Teeth Whitener Recipe

Everyone wants a whiter smile, but the cost of having your teeth professionally whitened can be astronomical. Over-the-counter teeth whiteners are also expensive and are loaded with chemicals that can be detrimental to your health. There is an alternative to expensive chemicals, and that is whitening your teeth with a natural recipe that can be made at

home. The recipe calls for sodium bicarbonate and hydrogen peroxide, which were shown in a study published in the Journal of the American Dental Hygiene Association to kill mouth bacteria, which can cause discoloration as well as cavities.

Step 1

Mix 2 tablespoons of hydrogen peroxide with enough baking soda to make a paste. Keep in an airtight container.

Step 2

Wet the bristles of a soft toothbrush with warm water. Dip the brush into the peroxide/baking soda paste and gently brush your teeth. Leave the paste on your teeth for 2 minutes.

Step 3

Hold the toothbrush under running water and rinse the mixture out of the brush. Now apply the wet toothbrush to your teeth and continue to rinse your teeth with the water and toothbrush until you have cleaned the paste off your teeth. Follow up with a final rinse of lukewarm water. Follow steps one through three twice a week.

Step 4

Take the cap off the hydrogen peroxide bottle and fill it with water. Put the water in your mouth, but do not swallow. Next, fill the cap with hydrogen peroxide and pour the capful of peroxide in your mouth. Again, do not swallow.

Step 5

Rinse your mouth for 1 minute with the diluted hydrogen peroxide. Spit out when finished. Perform this rinse (steps 4 and 5) twice daily.

CHAPTER 6: HOW TO GET RID OF BROWN SPOTS ON TEETH

Brown stains on your teeth are normally a result of coffee and cola consumption. Over time these beverages stain the teeth on the surface and these stains can enter cracks and crevices present on the enamel of the tooth. Even some medications can stain your teeth, according to Ronald I. Maitland, D.M.D in an excerpt from the "Doctor's Book of Home Remedies". One example of medication causing brown spots on your teeth is the antibiotic, tetracycline.

STEP 1

Brush your teeth after eating and drinking. Regular brushing will eliminate surface stains from your teeth. Using a whitening toothpaste may also help when applied two to three times a day for several months. Although it does not treat deeper staining, according to MayoClinic.com, it helps maintain whitening results from bleaching and will remove surface stains.

STEP 2

Mix together baking soda and peroxide to form a thick paste and apply to your toothbrush. Brush teeth with the paste to help polish away stains. The baking soda provides an exfoliating action as they hydrogen peroxide acts as a bleaching agent. According to Levin, be careful that you don't use too much hydrogen peroxide as this can cause burning and irritation.

STEP 3

Rinse your mouth with antibacterial mouthwash to reduce stained plaque. Stains are easily trapped in plaque and other build up that is common on your

teeth. Antibacterial mouthwash will kill and remove this plaque, according to the "Doctor's Book of Home Remedies".

STEP 4

Apply a tooth whitening strip or gel tray to your teeth once weekly, leaving on for up to 30 minutes. These kits work by bleaching the teeth with a hydrogen peroxide based solution. According to Daily Glow, some strips require treatment twice daily for up to two weeks before results are noticeable.

STEP 5

Opt for an in office dental bleaching at your dentist's office. Professional dental whitening is longer lasting and utilizes stronger hydrogen based gel. The gel is applied to your teeth and then exposed to a blue light to activate the whitening process according to Daily Glow. You are normally given a tray with hydrogen gel to take home with your for maintenance of your brighter smile.

CHAPTER 7: CONCLUSION

Hopefully you're feeling a lot better and with a boosted confidence thanks to our new found white smile. While I've done our part to give you a properly researched, balanced teeth whitening and cleaning
regimen, it's up to you to put it into action. Start achieving that perfect, sparkling smile that you deserve! Remember, consistency is key!

If you have any questions and/or requests (or if you like to be prompted before I release my next E-book), feel free to message me at : k.publishing2016@Gmail.Com

DISCLAIMER AND/OR LEGAL NOTICES

The information presented herein represents the view of the authors as of the date of publication. Because of the rate with which conditions change, the authors reserve the right to alter and update their opinion based on the new conditions. The report is for informational purposes only. While every attempt has been made to verify the information provided in this report, neither the authors nor their affiliates/partners assume any responsibility for errors, inaccuracies or omissions. Any slights of people or organizations are unintentional. If advice concerning legal or related matters is needed, the services of a fully qualified professional should be sought. This report is not intended as for use as a source of legal or accounting advice. You should be aware of any laws which govern business transactions or other business practices in your country and state. Any reference to any person or business whether living or dead is purely coincidental.